I0415187

A

Contents

B

C

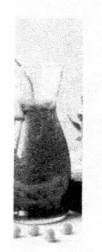

INTRODUCTION
TO SMOOTHIES

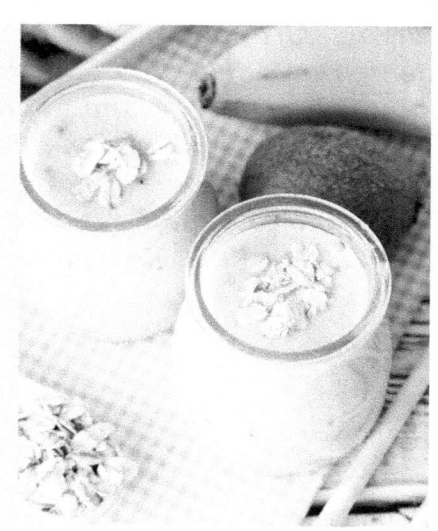

D

INTRODUCTION TO SMOOTHIES

Smoothies is an American name used for cold mixed fruit drinks and optional dairy products that are freshly prepared or sold as end products. Unlike fruit juices, the whole fruit and sometimes the bowl is processed into smoothies. The basis of the smoothies is, therefore, the fruit pulp or fruit puree, which is mixed with juices, water, milk, milk products or coconut milk, depending on the recipe, to obtain a creamy and creamy consistency.

Smoothies come in many different variations. Some smoothies only consist of fruit, such as pulp and juices. The banana is often a basic ingredient. The so-called "green smoothies" consist of water, leafy vegetables or garden or wild herbs and ripe fruit. There are also smoothies with yogurt, milk, ice cream, coconut milk or even supplements such as proteins, minerals or extra vitamins.

Just like their healthy counterparts, the juices and smoothies can be made from a wide range of organically grown, fresh fruits and vegetables. Smoothies, however, differ from juices in two ways:

1. They are made from whole fruit or vegetables
2. You can use many more healthy ingredients such as oats, nuts, seeds, herbs and many more natural supplements such as superfood.

Why Smoothie

Smoothies are a very good source of fiber
Fiber is the indigestible ingredients that can be
found in vegetable foods such as fruits, vegetables, grains, and legumes. Taking fibre is one
of the easiest and cheapest ways to prevent dis-
eases and maintain good health, as it helps to
rid the body of cellular waste and deadly toxins.
Water-soluble fibers lower cholesterol levels and
stabilize blood sugar. Water-insoluble fibres increase the number of stools and promote bowel
activity, remove toxic waste from the intestinal
wall and improve bowel health by reducing the
risk of diverticulosis and colorectal cancer.
Because smoothies are liquid or finely chopped
fruits and vegetables, smoothies contain both
water-soluble and water-insoluble fiber from the
plants. If you want more fibre, add psyllium, nuts,
seeds, boiled beans, bran or oatmeal to your
smoothie.
Fiber-rich vegetables and fruit are; Apples, orang-
es, berries, pears, figs, plums, broccoli, cauliflow-
er, Brussels sprouts, and carrots.
Smoothies are a healthy alternative to sweet soft
drinks.
This is because smoothies contain fiber and other ingredients that digest slowly, such as nuts,
seeds, milk, tofu or yogurt. These ingredients
saturate and satiate your hunger much more than
coffee or soft drinks.

Smoothies are an occasional meal replacement

In stressful times, smoothies are a quick meal replacement because they are high in nutrients. If you add small amounts of protein (such as hemp protein) and some cereal to your fruit/vegetable smoothie, you can upgrade your drink to a great meal replacement.

However, replacing all meals with long-term smoothies for several months is not a good idea, since people need a vast and wide variety of healthy natural foods. If other plants, e.g., Whole grains, beans, legumes, nuts, and seeds are omitted, you also limit the nutrients that your body can receive.

Breakfast and dinner are the best meals that can be replaced by a smoothie. Especially if you usually leave out your breakfast and then look for a quick meal during lunch because of the craving. Smoothies are an easy way to take medicinal herbs and supplements.

Older people or people who have had surgery can often take smoothies for a long time before they get solid food. You can mix your supplements with the ingredients of your smoothie.

You can increase your calorie intake by adding omega-3 rich oils and vegan protein sources. This is often the best way to improve the nutrition of old and malnourished people.

Medicinal herbs, tinctures, and tea can also be used as an ingredient in your smoothie. Healthy

supplements such as lecithin, bee pollen, vegan protein powder, Brussels sprouts can be added to the
blender together with the other ingredients.

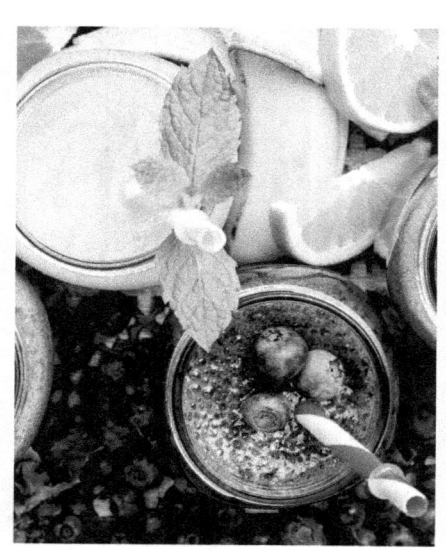

RECIPES

Banana, Raspberries, and Cacao

Ingredients
1 banana
30 g. raspberries
20 g. cacao powder
30 g. walnuts
200 g. cup water
200 g. cup ice

Blend until a nice smooth consistency

180 Cal

Pineapple, Cranberries and Baby Bok Choy

Ingredients
60 g. baby bok choy
110 g. pineapple
85 g. cranberries
1 orange - peeled
15g. ginger
200 g. water
200 g. cup ice

Blend until smooth

75 Cal.

Red Butter Leaf Lettuce and Oats

Ingredients
40 g. red butter leaf lettuce
1 apple - chopped
7 g. cinnamon
60 g. gluten-free oats
200 g. water
200 g. ice

Blend all ingredients and enjoy. Pour into glasses and serve.

96 Cal.

Carrots, Banana and Walnuts

Ingredients
140 g. carrots - chopped
1 banana - peeled
45 g. walnuts
5 g. cinnamon
200 g. water
200 g. ice

Put all ingredients into a blender. Blend until smoothie.

161 Cal.

Zucchini and Grapes

Ingredients
1 zucchini - chopped
115 g. grapes - stemmed
1 aprium - pitted
120 g. lemon - juice
45 g. almonds
200 g. water
200 g. ice

Put all ingredients into a blender. Blend until smoothie.

120 Cal.

Pear and Kiwi

Ingredients
40 g. swiss chard
1 pear - chopped
2 kiwis - peeled
2 g. tsp dried rose buds
200 g. water
200 g. ice

Blend all ingredients and enjoy.

109 Cal.

Strawberry and Yam

Ingredients
250 g. yams - scrubbed, chopped
170 g. strawberries - stemmed
1 orange - peeled
15 g. flaxseed
15 g. sunflower seeds
200 g. water
200 g. ice

Blend all ingredients and enjoy.

193 Cal.

Carrots Orange and Grape

Ingredients
140 g. carrots - chopped
1 orange - peeled
60 g. grape tomatoes
1 lemon - juiced
15 g sunflower seeds
200 g. water
200 g. ice

Put all ingredients into a blender. Blend until smoothie.

96 Cal.

Banana, Cherry, and Oat

Ingredients
1 banana - peeled
85 g. rhubarb
85 g. cherries
45 g. oats
200 g. water
200 g. ice

Put all ingredients into a blender. Blend until smoothie.

107 Cal.

Red Bell Pepper and Strawberries

Ingredients
140 g. red bell pepper - cored, seeded
85 g. strawberries
1 orange - peeled
15 g. flaxseed
200 g. water
200 g. ice
Put all ingredients into a blender. Blend until smoothie.
111 Cal.

Apple, Kiwi and Collard Greens

Ingredients
45 g. collard greens
1 apple - chopped
2 kiwis - peeled
15 g. chia seeds
200 g. water
200 g. ice

Blend all ingredients and enjoy.

118 Cal.

Avocado and Banana

Ingredients
45 g. swiss chard
1/2 avocado - pitted, peeled
1 banana - peeled
22 g. cacao powder
8 g. maca root powder
5 g. cinnamon
200 g. water
200 g. ice

Blend all ingredients and enjoy.

164 Cal.

Baby Spinach and Mango

Ingredients
45 g. baby spinach
110 g. mango - chopped
1 persimmon - chopped
30 g. coconut flakes
30 g. dried mulberries
200 g. water
200 g. ice

Blend all ingredients and enjoy.

115 Cal

Banana and Yellow Squash

Ingredients
1 banana - peeled
1 yellow squash - chopped
45 g. rolled oats
5 g. tsp cinnamon
30 g. almond butter
30 g. coconut cream
200 g. water
200 g. ice

Put all ingredients into a blender. Blend until smoothie.

233 Cal.

Swiss Chard, Persimmon and Cantaloupe

Ingredients
45 g. swiss chard
1 persimmon - chopped
140 g. cantaloupe
200 g. water
200 g. ice

Put all ingredients into a blender. Blend until smoothie.

100 Cal.

Baby spinach and Pear

Ingredients
45 g. baby spinach
1 pear - chopped
60 cranberries
200 g. water
200 g. ice

Put all ingredients into a blender. Blend until smoothie.

150 Cal.

Kiwi, Pear and Baby Spinach

Ingredients
45 g. baby spinach
1 pear - chopped
2 kiwis - peeled
15 g. rolled oats
200 g. water
200 g. ice

Blend all ingredients and enjoy.

120 Cal.

Carrots, Orange and Rhubarb

Ingredients
110 g. carrots - chopped
1 orange - peeled
52 g. rhubarb - chopped
200 g. water
200 g. ice

Put all ingredients into a blender. Blend until smoothie.

79 Cal.

Zucchini, Apple, and Strawberries

Ingredients
1 zucchini - chopped
1 apple - chopped
85 g. strawberries
1/2 lime - juiced
4 g. maqui berry powder
200 g. water
200 g. ice

Put all ingredients into a blender. Blend until smoothie.

81 Cal.

Baby Bok Choy and Plum

Ingredients
40 g. baby bok choy
1 plum - pitted
1 apple - chopped
4 g. chamomile
12 g. cashews
200 g. water
200 g. ice

Blend all ingredients and enjoy.

120 Cal.

Kiwi, Pear and Chia Seeds

Ingredients
40 g. mesclun mix
2 kiwis - peeled
1 pear - chopped
45 g. cashews
15 g. chia seeds
200 g. water
200 g. ice

Blend all ingredients and enjoy.

187 Cal.

Baby Kale and Cranberries

Ingredients
45 g. baby kale
85 g. cranberries
110 g. grapes
15 g.flaxseed
200 g. coconut water
200 g. ice

Put all ingredients into a blender. Blend until smoothie.
108 Cal.

Purple Sweet Potato and Pineapple

Ingredients
150 g. purple sweet potato - chopped
110 g. pineapple
1 pear - chopped
1 lime - juiced
5 g. maqui berry powder
200 g. water
200 g. ice

Blend all ingredients and enjoy.

102 Cal.

Apple, Cranberries, and Cucumber

Ingredients
50 g. collard greens
1 apple - chopped
60 g. cranberries
1 mini cucumber - chopped
5 g. dried hibiscus
5 g. flaxseed
200 g. water
200 g. ice

Put all ingredients into a blender. Blend until smoothie.

89 Cal.

Banana and Matcha

Ingredients
120 g. butternut squash - chopped
1 banana - peeled
5 g. pumpkin spice
5 g. matcha
200 g. water
200 g. ice

Blend until smooth.
91 Cal.

Almond Milk, Zucchini and Banana

Ingredients
50 g. collard greens
1 banana - peeled
1 zucchini - chopped
2 coconut flakes
60 g. cacao powder
200 g. almond milk
200 g. cup ice

Place all the ingredients in a blender. Blend on high speed until smooth
124 Cal.

Banana and Squash

Ingredients
1 banana - peeled
1 squash - chopped
45 g. rolled oats
5 g. lucuma powder
5 g. cinnamon
45 g. pumpkin seeds
200 g. water
200 g. ice

Combine all ingredients in a blender. Cover and blend.
125 Cal.

Baby Spinach, Orange and Banana

Ingredients
45 g. baby spinach
1 orange - peeled
1 banana - peeled
5 g. ginger
1 lemon - juiced
200 g. water
200 g. ice

Combine ingredients in a blender. Blend on medium speed until smooth.
Approximately 112 Calories.

Baby Spinach, Apple and Banana

Ingredients
45 g. baby spinach
1 apple - chopped
1 banana - peeled
5 g. cinnamon
15 g. sunflower seeds
200 g. water
200 g. ice

Blend all ingredients and enjoy.
Approximately 145 Calories.

Carrots, Orange and Banana

Ingredients
110 g. carrots - scrubbed, chopped
1 orange - peeled
1 banana - peeled
1 lime - juiced
30 g. goji berries
200 g. water
200 g. ice

Blend all ingredients and enjoy.
Approximately 123 calories

Baby Spinach, Pears,

Ingredients
40 g. baby spinach
2 pears - chopped
4 g. lucuma powder
30 g. coconut flakes
200 g. water
200 g. ice

Blend until smooth.
Approximately 164 calories.

Clementines, Cranberries, and Grapes

Ingredients
2 clementines - peeled
60 g. cranberries
120 g. grapes
45 g. rolled oats
15 g. hempseed
200 g. water
200 g. ice

Blend until smooth.
Approximately 115 calories

Baby Spinach, Banana and Oats

Ingredients
40 g. baby spinach
1 banana - peeled
1 container cinnamon applesauce
15 g. oats
45 g. pecans
200 g. water
200 g. ice

In a blender container, combine all ingredients.
Approximately 131 calories

Carrots, Pineapple and Kiwi

Ingredients
140 g. carrots - chopped
110 g. pineapple
1 kiwi peeled
45 g. cashews
15 g. flaxseed
200 g. water
200 g. ice

Place everything in a blender. Blend until SMOOTH!
Approximately 163 calories

Baby Spinach, Banana and Strawberries

Ingredients
45 g. baby spinach
1 banana - peeled
110 g. strawberries
22 g. cacao powder
200 g. almond milk
200 g. ice

In a blender container, combine all ingredients.
Approximately 107 calories

Pear, Orange, and Swiss Chard

Ingredients
40 g. swiss chard
1 pear - chopped
1 orange - peeled
5 g. lucuma powder
30 g. shredded coconut
200 g. water
200 g. ice

Put all ingredients into a blender. Blend until smoothie.

Approximately 107 calories

Nectarine, Orange and Chia

Ingredients
40 g. swiss chard
1 nectarine - pitted
1 orange - peeled
15 g. chia seeds
5 g. lucuma powder
200 g. water
200 g. ice

Blend until smooth.

Approximately 105 calories

Apple, Peach, and Lemon

Ingredients
40 g. swiss chard
1 apple - chopped
1 peach - pitted
50 g. rhubarb
5 g. ginger
1/2 lemon - juiced
45 g. walnuts
200 g. water
200 g. ice

In a blender container, combine all ingredients.

Approximately 150 calories

Honeydew, Pear and Yellow Squash

Ingredients
1 yellow squash - chopped
120 g. honeydew
1 pear - chopped
1/2 lemon - juiced
45 g. almonds
15 g. butterfly pea flower tea
200 g. water
200 g. ice

Put all ingredients into a blender. Blend until smoothie.
Approximately 160 calories

Lucuma, Pineapple, and Banana

Ingredients
40 g. collard greens
1 banana - peeled
120 g. pineapple
30 g. shredded coconut
5 g. lucuma
200 g. water
200 g. ice

Blend until smooth.

Approximately 93 calories

Grape tomatoes, Strawberries, and Orange

Ingredients
70 g. grape tomatoes
100 g. strawberries
1 orange - peeled
Small bunch basil leaves - stemmed
30 g. goji berries
30 g. pumpkin seeds
200 g. water
200 g. ice

In a blender container, combine all ingredients.
Approximately 119 calories

Sweet Potato, Mango and Orange

Ingredients
120 g. sweet potato - chopped
1/2 Ataulfo mango - pitted
1 orange - peeled
1 lime - juiced
1/2 avocado - pitted
30 g. coconut cream
200 g. water
200 g. ice

In a blender container, combine all ingredients.
214 calories

Plum, Yellow Squash and Acai Berry

Ingredients
1 yellow squash - chopped
1 plum - pitted
120 g. grapes
5 g. acai berry powder
45 g. almonds
200 g. water
200 g. ice

Blend all ingredients and enjoy.
142 calories

Carrots, Orange and Kiwi

Ingredients
120 g. carrots - chopped
1 orange - peeled
1 kiwi - peeled
45 g. cashews
200 g. water
200 g. ice

Blend all ingredients and enjoy.
Approximately 141 calories

Clementine, Kiwi, and Mangosteen

Ingredients
1 clementine - peeled
1 kiwi - peeled
120 g. pineapple
5 g. mangosteen powder
45 g. almonds
200 g. water
200 g. ice

In a blender container, combine all ingredients.

Approximately 134 calories

Baby Spinach, Pear and Cranberries

Ingredients
120 g. baby spinach
1 pear - chopped
60 g. cranberries
5 g. ginger
2 dates
45 g. walnuts
200 g. water
200 g. ice

Blend all ingredients and enjoy.

Approximately 160 calories

Collard Greens, Apple and Persian Cucumber

Ingredients
45 g. collard greens
1 apple - cored, chopped
60 g. cranberry
1 Persian cucumber - chopped
3 sprigs mint
15 g. dried hibiscus
15 g. flaxseed
200 g. water
200 g. ice

Put all ingredients into a blender. Blend until smoothie.
121 calories

Red Beets, Cranberries, and Apple

Ingredients
120 g. red beets - washed, chopped
50 g. cranberries
1 apple - chopped
1 lemon - juiced
15 g. flaxseed
200 g. water
200 g. ice

Put all ingredients into a blender. Blend until smoothie.
Approximately 110 calories

Purple Carrots, Banana and Walnuts

Ingredients
120 g. purple carrots
1 banana
5 g. maqui berry powder
45 g. walnuts
5 g. cinnamon
200 g. rice milk
200 g. ice

Blend until a nice smooth consistency
217 calories

Red Russian Kale, Pear, and Orange

Ingredients
40 g. oz red Russian kale
1 pear - chopped
1 orange - peeled
1 lime - juiced
200 g. cup water
200 g. cup ice

Put all ingredients into a blender. Blend until smoothie.
Approximately 112 calories

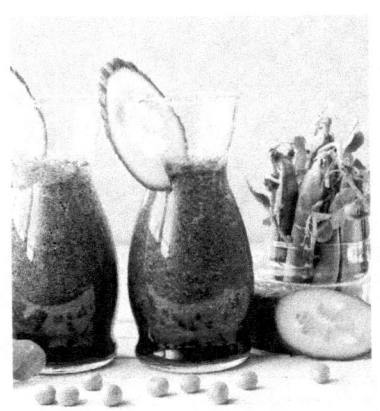

P.